THE HARDCORE FACTS

WHAT EVERY ATHLETE NEEDS TO KNOW TODAY ABOUT SPORTS NUTRITION FOR PEAK PERFORMANCE

MICHAEL P. ANGELILLO M.D.

iUNIVERSE, INC.
NEW YORK   BLOOMINGTON

The Hardcore Facts
What Every Athlete Needs To Know Today About
Sports Nutrition For Peak Performance

iUniverse books may be ordered through booksellers or by contacting:

iUniverse
1663 Liberty Drive
Bloomington, IN 47403
www.iuniverse.com
1-800-Authors (1-800-288-4677)

Because of the dynamic nature of the Internet, any Web addresses or links contained in this
book may have changed since publication and may no longer be valid. The views expressed
in this work are solely those of the author and do not necessarily reflect the views of the
publisher, and the publisher hereby disclaims any responsibility for them.

ISBN: 978-1-4401-5211-5 (sc)
ISBN: 978-1-4401-5212-2 (ebk)

Printed in the United States of America

iUniverse rev. date: 6/24/2009

ABOUT THE AUTHOR

Michael P. Angelillo M.D. is a board certified physician who has been in clinical practice for more than 20 years in South Florida were he resides with his family. He is an Internist with a subspecialty in Rheumatology and Sports Medicine. Dr. Angelillo had the distinct privilege to train under the auspices of Dr. Angelo Taranta, a world renoun Rheumatologist at Cabrini Medical Center in N.Y.C., responsible for his discovery work with Rheumatic Fever. As Co-Chief Resident in one of the largest teaching programs on the East Coast in New Jersey, Trenton Affiliated Hospitals affiliates of Hahnemann Medical College he taught medical residents in Internal Medicine. As a teacher, he has taught medical residents at New York University, Hospital For Joint Disease and Cornell Medical Center in New York. As and author, his is extensively published in various medical magazines and journals. Dr. Angelillo has also worked as an expert witness and medical consultant in South Florida. As an inventor, Dr. Angelillo invented the Arthrocentesis Kit, which has now become the standard of care in eliminating medical errors in the analysis of aspirated synovial fluid from affected joints. Dr. Angelillo has also been one of the team physicians for St. Thomas Aquinas High School Football Team, in Ft. Lauderdale which has won two consecutive State Championships in 2007 and 2008 and in 2008 was ranked number one high school football team in the entire nation. He has been affiliated with The American Medical Association, The Arthritis Foundation, The American College of Sports Medicine and The American College of Physicians. As being recognized in "Who's Who" for Professionals he was nominated, "One of the Most Intriguing People for 2003." The National Committee Physician Board has elected him the prestigious, " 2004 Physician of the Year Award."

DEDICATION

To my Mother and Father...

This book is dedicated to my father who passed away. He said, "trusting and believing in yourself gives one the inspiration needed to accomplish your goals in life."

To my mother, now in her mid-eighties says, "appreciate and love what you have today because what you have may not be loved or appreciated tomorrow."

CONTENTS

INTRODUCTION

Today more and more emphasis is being placed on how well you perform as an athlete. Many factors go into your abilities as an athlete. Your diet, how much sleep you get, genetics and hereditary, your training program, nutrition and conditioning program. A big part of your training should be placed on nutrition. Good nutrition should be a key part of your training program. What you do to provide the proper nutrients to your body could make the difference in your well-being, maintain desirable body weight, stay physically fit, and to establish optimum nerve to muscle reflexes thus enhancing your athletic ability.

Today athletes need to be bigger, faster and stronger. There is an ethical debate however over the concerns of using supplements to enhance athletic performance. The safety and legality of supplements are also concerns of the coaches and athletic trainers involved with the athlete. This apprehension to use supplements to enhance training and performance has lead to many coaches and trainers not recommending any supplement strategies. This is a mistake and may lead to a nutritional disadvantage for your athlete. **The purpose of this book is to provide the latest nutritional strategies that are safe, legal and effective for enhancing performance in today's athlete to give them the edge needed for maximal performance.**

Nutrients like proteins, carbohydrates, fats, vitamins, minerals, and water provide the essentials for great athletic performance. A lack of one of these nutrients will put your body at a disadvantage for optimum performance.

Other essential supplements will be discussed in detail in this book which will give you the facts about how these nutrients and supplements can be used to get the best results to enhance your athletic performance.

The information presented in this book will present facts about supplements and nutrients that have proven to enhance your athletic ability. This book will not go over workout routines. Before reading this book ask yourself, **"Why** should I not have the advantage of knowing all that is to know about supplements and nutrients to practically help me succeed as an athlete?"

For the first time by reading this book a summary of condensed up to date knowledge of critically proven facts about supplements and nutrition that apply to everyday training will be revealed to give an athlete the advantage for your peak performance.

CHAPTER 1
PRE-WORK OUT/GAME MEAL

One of the most important things on game day is to be prepared by your pre-game meal. You should know that days prior to your event you should already start the process of adequate hydration. Always drink plenty of fluids with your pre-game meal. There are certain do's and dont's to a pre-game meal. This book will provide you factual data about pre-game meals which you may or may not be aware of.

For instance an easy digestible meal should only be considered. This means a meal with **FATS** and **OILS** should be avoided due to slow digestible qualities. Foods that contain **SUGAR** should be avoided. These types of foods will cause swings in blood sugar levels and result in low blood sugar and less energy. Avoid foods and drinks that contain **CAFFIENE.** Caffiene stimulates the body to increase urine output, which leads to dehydration problems. A pre-game meal prior to your event should be ingested no later than **three hours before a game.**

The golden rule to a pre-game meal is to increase the amount of glycogen, or animal starch, stored in the liver and muscle tissue. Scientific studies have collaborated and said if you can saturate your liver and muscle tissue with enough stored glycogen you have then accomplished your goal with a pre-game meal. At the start of your sports competition event you have accomplished getting as much glycogen in the liver and muscle tissue to carry you through the sports or work out routine.

What should you eat pre-game? **Scientific data states a meal which contains the STARCHES is the most desirable meal.**

By eating a high **Carbohydrate** meal with exercise has been proven scientifically to increase the body's stores of glycogen in the liver and muscle tissue. Foods which have been shown to accomplish this for a pre-game meal include pancakes, rice and noodles. Other foods mutually beneficial are, spaghetti, potatoes (mashed, boiled or baked) not french fries. **Starchy vegetable,** rolls, muffins, crackers, quick breads, bagels will give you sufficient glycogen stores. **Cereals**, oatmeal (if not high in sugar). Soups, and bouillon are good. **Fruits, Milk products** low in fat are good too.

In looking at past experiences regarding pre-game meals the problem is that team meals are consisting of mostly protein. **Eating a diet high in protein as part of a pre-game meal is also not recommended.** Routine protein could be obtained by eating normal meals with protein. Scientific data now shows that a high protein meal can actually cause a loss of appetite, diarrhea, dehydration, and stress on the kidneys.

Try to break up your meals game day by eating frequent times a day. Six times a day is said to be perfect for digestion. It is preferred that you eat every three-four hours to give you body time to digest and store your efforts. Most importantly remember to consume fluids. I will further elaborate on how much to drink in the next chapter of water.

CHAPTER 2

WATER

Athletes have a special need for water. Participating in Sports like football, track, and field, baseball you burn a lot of Calories or food energy. During exercise substantial amount of Fluid are lost due to perspiration and to a lesser extent water vapor Lost during breathing. Energy is released as heat. Water can keep you from overheating. Sweating and evaporation from the pores of your skin can cool you down. If water is lost in the cooling process this can be very dangerous as your body can then overheat. It is estimated that loosing 2% of your body's water can hurt your actual performance. Just a 5% loss can cause heat exhaustion and a 7% lose can cause a heat stroke and death!

By the time you are thirsty, you have already lost approximately 1-2% of your body water. This has been shown to hurt your overall performance. If you wait to drink because you are thirsty it will then take approximately 24 hrs. to replenish your body water. To perform your best, all sweat/fluid lost during activity should be replaced.

How much you should drink has now been determined to depend on the size of the athlete, the intensity of the sport, the relative humidity, temperature. **According to the American College of Sports Medicine, a guideline during physical activity is to drink 20-40 ounces per hour of a non-carbonated beverage. Drink 5-10 ounces of fluid every 15-20 minutes. (An ounce of fluid equals approximately one gulp.)**

Ideally for best performance studies have shown that peek performance is reached when you are fully hydrated when you begin your activity or exercise.

Two hours prior to physical activity you should drink at least two cups (16 ounces) of fluid which is non-carbonated, little carbohydrate and no caffeine. This will give your body energy to burn. Gatorade Thirst Quencher has the optimal amount of carbohydrate (14g/8oz.) and sodium

(110mg/8oz.) which has proven re-hydration benefits over water alone.

Research shows that flavored fluids, and lightly sweetened that contain some sodium help stimulate voluntary drinking more than water alone. Fruit juices or non-diet soft drinks have approximately twice the amount of sugar of sports drinks and if consumed during exercise slow absorption and cause cramping or stomach aches. To check your hydration status check the color of your urine. **In general the lighter the color of your urine the better you are hydrated!**

CHAPTER 3

PROTEIN

Protein is a necessary nutrient needed for maintaining normal health. There have been many claims made in the literature about the use of protein and how much protein is required for an athlete. At one time, it was believed that muscle-building exercise increased dietary protein needs. But research has shown that increasing basic foods to meet your increased energy needs will supply more than enough protein. It has been disputed in the long distance runner that extra amounts of protein could be utilized if needed. Eating high –protein diets or taking protein supplements may prove harmful and may lead to loss of appetite, diarrhea, dehydration, and stress on the kidneys. Besides, extra protein is expensive.

Today it is estimated that athletes take in more protein than required. **The fact is that your protein intake should be no greater than 2grams/kg. of body weight per day** to enhance muscle growth. An example is if a male athlete weighted 200lbs. or 90kg. his intake of protein for the day would be approximately 200grams of protein. This intake should be of course taken in multiple (six) meals per day. **Note the scientific evidence reveals that added protein intake does not enhance recovery.**

High protein diets increase the risk of certain cancers. On the market today you will find many types of protein supplements. Whey, Casein, Egg, Soy proteins are available. For the athlete in training which protein should you buy? **The scientific evidence supports Whey Protein.** Whey protein is far superior to any other type of protein. Whey has a complete amino acid profile for muscle building and is the fastest digesting protein source on the market.

When should you take protein shakes or supplements? Scientific evidence shows that the morning, immediately after a work out session and bedtime are the most efficient and beneficial times to take protein supplements.

CHAPTER 4
CARBOHYDRATES

Carbohydrate supplements are used in sports activities to provide energy and are useful before, during and after a training session or activity performance. How much carbohydrate should one have? **As a general rule scientific evidence has proven that the body can only process about 60 grams of carbohydrate per hour or (1gm/kg).** Carbohydrates consist of starch, sugars and sugar alcohols and organic acids. All carbohydrates can be classified as monosaccharides, oligosaccharides or polysaccharides.

Carbohydrates are the main source of energy for all body functions. Carbohydrates are used for energy storage. The highest source of carbohydrates are found in foods such as breads, beans, milk, popcorn, potatoes, cookies, spaghetti, corn and cherry pie. Glucose is the main sugar metabolized by the body for energy. It fuels the brain and muscles. Only mono-saccharides, glucose, fructose and galactose are absorbed in humans.

Galactose can be converted into glucose when needed for energy. Fructose can be converted into glucose in the liver and intestines. Glycogen is a polysaccharide made up of repeated glucose units. Glycogen can be converted into energy to sugar for the muscle cells. An athlete which requires a rapid replacement of carbohydrates stores should eat or drink as soon as possible after exercise.

You should choose a carbohydrate which has a high glycemic index. Carbohydrates with higher indexes are absorbed in the gastrointestinal track faster, for faster recovery. A more rapid rise in blood sugar will take place for a faster recovery if a high gycemic index carbohydrate is used. **For fast recovery after a hard workout replace and eat 1-1.2 grams of carbohydrate/kg of body weight each hour for the first 4 hours. If much high endurance exercise is anticipated or a much longer workout period then a replacement of up to 10grams of carbohydrate/ kg of body weight is required.**

Note liquid and solid forms of carbohydrate are equally effective in replenishing glycogen. High Glycemic Index foods include corn flakes, baked potato, watermelon, croissants, white bread, Rice Krispies and Sport Drinks which contain a Gycemic index above 75.

CHAPTER 5

ANABOLIC STERIODS

Agencies like the National Football League (NFL), the National Collegiate Athletic Association (NCAA), and the International Olympic Committee (IOC) have banned the use of steroids from sports. Anabolic Steroids are hormones that help the body build muscle tissue which increases muscle mass. This is similar to the hormone testosterone.

When taking steroids the muscle tissue grows, producing larger and stronger muscle. An athlete who uses steroids must understand there is a risk for various increase in cancers. **Steroids have now been proven to develop cholesterol patterns associated with coronary heart disease, obstructing blood vessels which has lead to stroke. Regarding the heart there is now proven data that there is an associated**

increase in blood pressure with elevated cholesterol.

In the liver there are early signs of liver impairment. Tumors and reported Peliosis Hepatitis (which are blood-filled cysts which rupture and cause liver failure) have been reported. Regarding the skeleton, stunted growth now is evident, caused by premature closing of cartilage growth plates in adolescents.

The skin can exhibit striae (stretch marks). Increase of acne has been evident now occurring as early as the first week of the onset of steroid use. An increase of Hepatitis B or C, and HIV has occurred since needles are being shared. Now a proven fact are mood swings, depression, aggressive violent behavior and psychotic episodes occur. **Newly reported now is an addiction to steroid use**.

Specifically in men, infertility, sterility, prostate enlargement, breast enlargement, painful erections, shrinkage of testicles, increase levels of estrogens and abnormal sperm production, and prostate cancer. In females, increase in cervical and endometrial cancer, increase risk of osteoporosis, altered sex drive, sterility, birth defects in children, changes in fat distribution, growth of facial hair, deeper voice, breast reduction, clitoral enlargement and most commonly menstrual irregularity.

Steroids can be injected or taken orally. Steroids that are injected stay in your system longer. Oral steroids typically stay in the body for several weeks where injectable steroids stay in your body and can be detected for several months. Steroids that are taken orally put a burden on your liver. **Note: there has been an increase in contamination, mislabeling of steroids.** This has led to an increase in side effects.

Before taking or considering taken steroids you should ask yourself can steroids improve athletic performance? The facts are that steroids will increase bulk muscle, strength, but cannot improve athletic skill, and agility and decreases the cardiovascular capacity! Also it is now a fact that steroid use will decrease recovery time from injuries and slows down the process of healing time.

More important facts about steroids are that there has been an increase in suicide, homicide, heart attacks, cancers and death. In addition steroids cause tolerance which has lead the chronic user to increase dosage.

Finally, if you know someone needing help from steroid use give them or call for them your local Council on Alcohol and Drug Abuse Center in your city.

CHAPTER 6

HUMAN GROWTH HORMONE

Human Growth Hormone or HCG is now the most widely used supplement in the United States by athletes. Today doctors can legally prescribe growth hormone injection for those teenagers who have certain hormone or growth problems to help them grow normally.

Growth Hormone starts to decline in the body as we grow older. A fact is after the age of 30 years old GH declines by 25 % every decade. By the time you are 60 years old you have 25 % of the original hormone.

Growth hormone was discovered in the 1920's and was isolated in the form of somatotropin in 1956. Growth hormone is present between the ages of 20 and 30 at the rate of 500 micrograms at any time in the blood. It is produced in the anterior pituitary gland under the stimulus of the hypothalmus.

The proven facts about growth hormone to date is that HGH promotes and increases the synthesis of new protein tissues, such as muscle recovery or repair. This is how new muscle is built. Recent research suggest its involvement in the metabolism of body-fat and its conversion to energy sources. Growth hormone will increase lean mass. It has proven to improve REM sleep. HGH produces more energy. It will build stronger bones. **The facts are that HGH in limited doses has shown no side effects.**

A very important question to ask yourself is how can I increase my growth hormone naturally? Growth hormone production can be manipulated. By putting the body under extreme stress (training) you can stimulate growth hormone. Most common way is to lift weights. Energy consuming events and long periods of physical exhaustion are keys in releasing more growth hormone.

This occurs because these catabolic states require extra protein synthesis and in case of lack of energy, fat metabolization makes up for glycogen depletion. **The general rule of thumb**

is never train longer than 45 minutes because GH tapers off and cortisol production sets in.

Rest is another important factor. It is a fact that 75 % of your daily HGH output is produced while sleeping in REM sleep. The most HGH can be manufactured with close to 7-8 hours of sleep.

The most important factor to stimulate more growth hormone naturally is to make sure you are digesting amino acids (Arginine, Ornithine, Glutamine, Glycine, Lysine). Other dietary sources are Vitamin C, Vitamin B3 and anti-oxidants.

CHAPTER 7

DEHYDROEPIAND-ROSTERONE (DHEA)

DHEA called dehydroepiandrosterone is a hormone which is produced naturally from cholesterol in the adrenal glands of males and females. What has made this supplement popular in athletic sports is that is the precursor to the sex hormone testosterone. The production now is noted to peak in your mid 20's and actually declines in the early 30's. DHEA has noted to drop by 90% by the time you are 70 years old. Originally the Food and Drug Administration classified DHEA as a drug. By 1994 it was reclassified as a dietary supplement obtainable without a prescription.

Looking at all the factual data it is unclear how the hormone works in the body and what it does. There is overwhelming evidence that over the past 30 years of study DHEA increase energy, enhance sex drive, and improved ability to deal with stress and well being. This data was on 50mg of DHEA daily for 3 consecutive months. Studies done on rodents have shown a clear benefit from preventing cancer, heart disease, and AIDS. It has also shown to beneficial in fighting of viral infections and obesity. DHEA now has shown to have anti-aging properties. New facts about DHEA have shown an increase in the risks of male prostate cancer and in women endometrial and breast cancer because of the related increase in testosterone and estrogen levels.

In the sports medicine world DHEA is converted to androstenedione and then testosterone. The hormone then has two chances to become estrogen-estrone from androstenedione, and estradiol from testosterone. It ultimately increases estrogen levels and testosterone.

Today DHEA in the U.S Senate (S.762) has been classified as an anabolic steroid and a controlled substance. It has now been referred to the Senate Judiciary Committee for further ruling.

CHAPTER 8

CREATINE

Creatine will now be promoted as a muscular performance enhancer, and there is scientific evidence to support this. **The goal of Creatine supplementation is to increase muscle phosphocreatine and make more ATP available to fuel the working muscles.** Creatine occurs naturally in foods like meat and fish. Creatine is also manufactured by the body in the liver, kidneys, and pancreas. Extra creatine ingested is stored in the muscle which is believed to give athletes their boost in energy.

A 70kg adult about a 154lb. adult has about 120 grams of creatine in their muscles and everyday about 2 grams are utilized daily. Scientific evidence reveals about half of this is replaced by the diet and half is synthesized endogenously. Creatine is eliminated from the body by the kidneys as creatine or as creatinine.

In has now been shown that scientifically the power athletes who are using creatine benefited their performance because of high intensity workouts. The endurance athletes like runners did not benefit from creatine intake, instead it was shown to cause muscle cramps and tears. **The facts are Creatine will improve high power performance during a series of repetitive high power output exercise sessions but does not increase indurance or exert an anabolic effect.** Short term side effects, creatine taken for less than two weeks failed to show side effects. Over two week period approximately 20 grams per day can cause diarrhea, weight gain, abdominal pain, dehydration. Kidney failure has also been reported. It also increases your risk for heat illness. There is usually a 5-10 loading dose for creatine in the body before maintaining a creatine level daily in the muscle tissue.

CHAPTER 9

FAT BURNERS /
THERMOGENESIS

When talking about supplements in sports medicine one can not leave out one supplement which is on the rise in athletes. Fat burners are a dietary supplement claimed to accelerate fat loss. If you survey the commercial products promoted as fat burners many contain ephedrine alkaloids derived from the herb Ephedra. This group of alkaloids belong to the group of drugs called stimulants. These supplements are on The World Anti-Doping Agency Prohibited List. **On April 12, 1994 the FDA ruled and banned supplements which contain ephedra.**

Ephedra-containing supplements accelerate weight loss, but have damaging effects on the cardio-vascular, nervous, and thermoregulatory systems in our bodies. For nutritionist and those assisting with the development of athletic performance a fat burner is a product directed at the utilization of stored fats and their conversion into free fatty acids in the production of energy to fuel the body. It is now known that the body can conserve carbohydrates and at the same time consume fats. This process is now known as thermogenesis. **Fat burners have now been proven to work by raising our core body temperature of 1degree accelerating metabolism**. Fat burners can be also composed of guarana, coffee, and the ingredient bitter orange which all can suppress appetite.

By taking fat burners one is increasing the bodies metabolism which burns up more calories. Although these supplements have shown to burn more calories one has to consider the side effects associated with its constant use.

CHAPTER 10
VITAMIN SUPPLEMENTS

In sports medicine it is important to state that vitamins play a significant role in overall peak performance. **Vitamins are the most commonly used dietary supplements among various athletic groups**. Athletes who are deficient in vitamins are at particular risk for poor performance. This has been shown to be true of the younger athlete who does not adhere to a well balanced diet.

The scientific facts today reveal vitamin deficiencies can impair exercise performance. Studies have shown that a daily intake of less than one-third of the RDA for several of the B vitamins (B1, B2, and B6) and Vitamin C, even when other vitamins are supplemented in the diet, leads to a significant decrease in

overall performance and endurance in less than four weeks.

Vitamins function in the human body as metabolic regulators for exercise and performance. For example many of the B-complex vitamins are involved in processing carbohydrate and fats for energy production. B-vitamins also are essential to help form hemoglobin in red blood cells, a major determinant of oxygen delivery to the muscles during aerobic endurance exercise.

One widely used vitamin today is **Niacin.** It is used to treat and lower cholesterol. Niacin has now been proven to influence fat metabolism which block the release of free fatty acids from adipose tissue which then increases carbohydrate metabolism leading to the depletion of muscle glycogen. **Researches have now documented that excess Niacin vitamins which are used to treat cholesterol lowering will actually impair aerobic endurance and performance. B1, B6, B12 affects the formation of serotonin a neurotransmitter involved in relaxation.**

New data confirms that in dosages ranging from 60 to 200 times the RDA increase fine motor control and performance. This data has been shown to increase the performance in sports with pistol shooting which uses fine motor control.

Choline if found naturally in a variety of foods and its RDA is grouped with the B vitamins. Research has shown that Choline is involved in the formation of acetylcholine which is a neurotransmitter whose reduction in the nervous system contributes to fatigue. Facts about Choline show that marathon runners show low levels of plasma Choline after a race. **Research and new data show that replacing Choline will reverse our symptoms of fatigue.** This is a critical fact in sports medicine and recovery for the athlete. Dosages and replenishment have still not been worked out.

Vitamin C supplement has been shown to improve physical performance in vitamin C deficient subjects only. Vitamin C supplementation does not enhance physical performance in well nourished individuals.

Vitamin E has been shown to enhance oxygen utilization during exercise at high altitude but not at sea level conditions. There is no effect on training, performance or post exercise recovery in athletes.

CoQ10, ubiquinone is an antioxidant which improves oxygen uptake in the mitochondria of the heart, and has been utilized to treat heart disease. This could ultimately prove to be beneficial to improve human performance. Studies have now concluded that taking CoQ10 have improved muscle damage in cycling.

Preventing muscle tissue damage during exercise training may help optimize the training effect and eventual competitive sport edge in overall competition. **It has now been concluded that supplementation with antioxidant vitamins has favorable effects on lipid peroxidation and exercise induced muscle damage and recommend vitamin supplementation to athletes who perform regular heavy exercise.** Antioxidants, Vitamin C, and Vitamin E can prevent muscle tissue damage by decreasing the exercise induced increase ratio for lipid peroxidation. Vitamin E is suggested at 100-200 milligrams.

One important fact is that athletes involved in heavy training need more vitamins, such as Thiamin, Riboflavin and B6 because they are involved in energy production. Note that athletes may be at risk for vitamin deficiency, such as those in weight controlled sports and those who for one reason or another do not eat a well balanced diet.

CHAPTER 11

WHAT'S NEW FOR PEAK PERFORMANCE

Today anyone who is serious about physical performance is looking for an edge which is often in the form of a practical and safe supplement to improve parameters of athletic performance and achievement. When finding the right performance enhancer can be a challenge. Remember, what works for one person may not necessarily provide the same benefits for another.

Herbal Boosters like Ginseng has only recently been discovered by athletes as a way of strengthening the immune system and providing extra energy. Ginseng must be taken for several weeks before its effects are likely to be felt. One form of Ginseng is **Ciwujia also known as Siberian** Ginseng. Numerous studies have shown that during exercise Ciwujia burns fat rather than carbohydrates, which translates into longer workouts with less soreness.

Another remarkable Chinese supplement with athletic applications is **Cordycepts Sinensis, also called Cordyceps Mycelia a fungus. This has been shown to increase endurance and lung capacity while decreasing recovery time and protect against infection.**

The two supplements that build both strength and muscle mass are Tribulus Terrestris and Yohimbe Bark Extract.

These raise testosterone production naturally, without harming the liver or kidneys resulting in increase energy and endurance. HMB (beta hydroxyl-beta methylbutyrate) is an amino acid metabolite which supports the body's ability to minimize the breakdown of protein following intense exercise. This causes HMB to increase muscle mass and strength. In addition, this supplement helps to speed up the loss of body fat, as well as recovery from exercise induced muscle damage and post- workout soreness.

Pyruvate has been shown to improve athletic endurance by helping to remove glucose from the blood circulating into muscle cells.

Pyruvate also helps to promote weight loss in overweight people by boosting metabolism and increase endurance.

L- Carnitine is necessary for releasing energy from fat. This decreases the need for carbohydrate as the energy source. This nutrient helps transport fatty acids into the mitochondria, making exercise more productive. Studies have documented that L- Carnitine also decreases muscle soreness after exercise.